Cookie Boobs
My Cancer Journey
A.Lady

Teresa

Freindship
is never a thing of
time but quality

love you
Mom

Cookie Boobs

Copyright © 2023 by A. Lady

ISBN: 978-1-7388574-0-1

Edited by Dennis Doty

http://www.dennisdotywebsite.com/editing.html

Cover by: Lisa Pederson

FIRST EDITION: February 2023

Dedicated to Everyone who has had to do something really scary and still took that first step.

Warrior
Noun

1. Shows great courage and perseverance
2. One with the willpower to overcome any struggle
3. Badass

Monday

I have Breast Cancer.

It took me over a week and starting to see a counselor before I could say that without having a meltdown or a panic attack or both at once. I hate the ownership of "I have." But I can't reverse it either, "Breast Cancer has me" is even less acceptable and wrong. It doesn't have me, and I'm evicting it ASAP. I'm not sure what to say yet, but I will think of a way to say it without it taking my power, my strength from me.

Making the phone calls to my family and friends was really hard. I had to tell them I had cancer. And it is so scary to them as well as me. Lots of questions I can't answer yet. But lots of love too. Supportive words, plans made to be there when I go for surgery or whatever the plan becomes.

It started with a routine mammogram. Then, the call to return for another mammogram and an ultrasound. I called my doctor to let her know and she immediately took my off my HRT (hormone replacement therapy) medication in case there is something there and it is growing from the hormones. She told me that when the results come in that I will be her last appointment of the day so we will have time to talk; good results or bad. Thankfully they only had to squish one poor boob again! After the ultrasound, the radiologist and I talked. He told me there is a shadow that looks granular so they want to do a biopsy of the area. The tech drew a large black dot with a felt marker on the side of my breast to mark where the biopsy would be. I hate looking at the black smear when I shower so, I decided to take this back, to not give into the fear. I took a pink highlighter and drew looping petals around it and turned it into the centre of a daisy. Now I have a flower that makes me smile instead of a menacing black spot. Needles freak me out and here I am about to get a really big needle taking tissue samples! I tell the tech if they would just tell me I'm doing fine and not that they are putting the freezing in that would be great. I concentrate on breathing through my diaphragm so I don't move my breast any more than necessary. The tech warned me that the biopsy needle would push down and sound like a stapler. When I was laying the way they needed me with the sterile drape on, the procedure started. Well, it started after they laughed at the sight of my flower and told me they had never seen anyone turn the ugly mark into something fun and pretty. The freezing wasn't bad and the biopsy needle did sound like a big stapler. Since I knew what to expect it took a lot of the scariness away. And now the waiting begins. The results will be back in eight to ten days. Finally, I get the call from my doctor's office to come in at end of the day. The waiting has been so hard but the results are finally in and they are positive for cancer. 19 days from my routine mammogram and my world is tilted on its axis.

Tuesday

It was a cold room. Not in temperature, but in atmosphere. The kind of room that makes you want a sweater on the hottest day, not for the warmth but for the comfort. There was a marble-faced, unlit fireplace against one wall. Drapes gave the illusion of windows where there were none. The floor was polished stone. There were two chairs in the room, the kind that, although padded and fabric covered, demanded an upright posture on them. Each chair had a small table beside it big enough for a cup and a small plate. In one chair sat Cancer, disdain and arrogance plainly showing in its every line. It watched a small child who was crying and screaming as she ran around the room. "You can't leave you know," it said. "You are trapped here with me." The child ignored it—beating on the walls, looking for a door where none existed.

As Cancer plucked another delicacy from the plate and popped it into its mouth, a door appeared in the wall where moments before there was none. The child was spent, laying in a heap on the floor. A woman came into the room. Sparing barely a glance for Cancer, she went to the keening heap on the floor and sat beside her. "Come here." She said as she scooped the child into her lap. "Come sit with me." The woman wrapped the softest, warmest blanket around the child and hugged her close.

"Why are you crying?" asked the child. "Because I am scared too," said the woman. "And because I was scared, I walled Cancer up I this room. But I didn't realize I had walled you up in here too, and I'm so sorry for that. I won't leave you alone again." The woman looked at Cancer as she spoke to the child. "Cancer and I will have to talk. It knows it's not welcome here; but it also knows that even though I can't make it leave yet, it's confined to this room, so you are safe to go, and it can't follow."

Cancer stares back and with a faint nod, acknowledges what the woman has said as it plucks another tender morsel from the plate, the threat unspoken hanging in the air between them that, if Cancer decided to move from the chair, there was nothing the woman could do to stop it—Yet. So, the woman rocked and comforted the child who, feeling safer, fell asleep in her arms as silent tears drip down her face.

Wednesday

"You are a Liar and a Thief. A Destroyer of Innocence. You sneak in through the little cracks in the dark and invade through deception and deceit. You are not welcome here Trespasser and Squatter. And I will use everything at my disposal to make sure you are evicted and permanently barred from ever entering again."

"You are welcome to try," replied Cancer. "But you know that, even if you take me from my current chair in your house and put me outside, you will always wonder if I will find a new way in, or if I left a little something behind. And every time you look at the disfigurement on your body—the damage done to remove me—you will know I was there and may return as I like."

"That scar will be a badge of honor. Scars show what a person has battled and overcome. I will survive you, and

I will have the marks to prove it. I am a strong woman. A warrior who goes to battle daily for those around me. Today I go to battle for myself, and those around me battle with me. I will defeat you. You will lose this battle, and I will stand with my sword at your neck, my foot on your back.

Cancer wasn't so arrogant and sure of itself. It shrank down a bit in the chair. Instead of plucking small bits from the dish, it grabbed handfuls, gulping them down, growing bloated and gross—Showing its true face. No aristocrat here. Rather a cheap thief who wore a cloak of illusion and power.

Thursday

Had my surgery consult and I have decided to get a mastectomy.

The entire time I was in the appointment with the surgeon I was thinking I would just get a lumpectomy. Get the offending area removed and keep my breasts. Then he told me that cancer in the milk duct was the most common one for women. And even though I hadn't consciously made the decision, when he asked me what I wanted to do, Mastectomy was what came out of my mouth. But it felt right, so I stuck with it, because there is a milk duct in both sides. I do not want to wonder if it's going to reappear in the other breast, like one ear cocked for the other shoe to drop.

The doctor's office put me in touch with the Women's Breast Health Clinic. This was an amazing group of people. They contacted me with every appointment to go over what to expect with the appointment and also after to see if I had any questions. They were a wonderful resource, and it was so good to know that I had a single number I could call to organize and make sense of what was happening and the next steps. Without them this journey would have been so much harder.

Friday

When you hide from pain it only gets worse. Best to deal with it as it comes so you can learn and grow from it. Not be swamped by it when it gets too big.

People say, "My troubles seem paltry compared to yours."

"You are so kind to help out with this, with all you're going through."

Perspective – Hurt is hurt. And it should be honored and recognized with empathy and compassion. My hurt is no more nor less than yours. It's just different.

Yes, I am going through this battle, but that doesn't mean that what is happening with you is irrelevant. And why would I suddenly stop being kind just because I have cancer? It's a disease, not a personality transplant. And it is important to not allow cancer to rule my life and my actions or let things become "all about me" or be colored by the fact that I have cancer. That's the wrong mentality, and I am all about the fight to win.

My Dad was a boxer. And he taught me how to box when I was little. But the most important lesson he taught me was to make the first hit count because you might not get a second one. And that is why I am getting a Bilateral Mastectomy. Both breasts are going. No more breasts, no more milk ducts for cancer to hide in.

Saturday

I am cautious who I tell about this. I don't want to be gossiped about or have snoopy/invasive questions asked. I have told my family and the friends that I know will support me; not the ones I will have to support instead. I need my strength and need strong people I can lean on with me to make this battle successful.

Sunday

I am planning to get a Bilateral Mastectomy. I will not chance it coming back in the other breast. On the up-side, the surgeons will be able to do re-construction (hopefully from my own body) at the same time as they take away the invaded tissue.

Bilateral Mastectomy. This means the surgeon will cut off both my breasts. In their entirety. The breasts that I have had since I was seven years old, in a training bra. The breasts that fed my babies will be no more. I need to consider this for a while. There will be grieving for what I am losing but also relief for it to be finished.

When I look at myself, I just see me. One breast slightly smaller than the other, like most women. That's the one the cancer was found in. In the milk duct. By making the choice to have both breasts removed at once, I am removing the risk of cancer moving to the other side, into the other milk duct.

The positives I am taking from this surgery are: No more milk ducts for the cancer to hide in, 'perky' (even if that's the only perky thing about me) symmetrical new breasts, they should be able to reconstruct them from my stomach tissue which means a tummy tuck too.

And I am holding on to those things with all my strength. Because this is very scary s**t. And if I dwell on it too much, I will be paralyzed by it.

Another Sunday

Hope is like Air. We need both to survive. If we have no hope the spirit suffocates under despair. On the days when I feel despair/sorrow covering me like a heavy wet blanket making it hard to move or even breathe; I take a moment; sometimes hiding in the bathroom if I'm at work, to just breathe. To feel the air filling my lungs, my heartbeat under my hand and think about one little thing that makes me happy. The birdsong when I stepped outside. The sound of the rain on the roof. How cozy my blankets were when I woke up this morning. Just one little thing. And then another little thing until the little things build up to a big pile of joy and I have hope again that I can do this. No one can fight 24/7. We must take time to rest, to eat, to connect with our people. So, today I am going to get dressed, go for a walk and smile at anyone I meet. I will buy a tea at the corner store and walk home. I won't rush there or back. I will take my time and look for joy and hope along the way.

Monday

Sometimes the feelings I have are all jumbled up like a skein of wool that a kitten has gotten into. All tangled in a horrible mess. And the ball is full of knots and loops. And the whole thing is made of thin shiny wire with sharp barbs and the centre of it glows like it's full of electricity. Snapping and crackling. Other times, it's a lump like a stone, dull and heavy. Going to the counsellor has helped untangle the feelings and thoughts to I can look at them for what they are and deal with them accordingly.

Tuesday

It makes me angry the way people sometimes refer to how things are – everything is colored by the cancer. I was talking to someone about struggling with life sometimes. And she said she could understand why I would be struggling. I told her I've always struggled, the same as everyone else. Good days and bad. There's nothing new there just because of the cancer. *Now* I'm brave? Why? Because I'm not wailing and raging against the injustice of it? Because I am putting a good face on it? Any crying I do is in the privacy of my home. I am not a spectacle nor am I a victim. It's not like I chose this path. I'm just doing the best I can with the hand I've been given. S**t happens, sometimes you have to tip your head back and wade with your nose just above it. But you don't stand in it, and you certainly don't lay down and drown in it. Sometimes when you move forward it is giant leaps, and other times it is the tiniest of steps. But you still move forward. And you celebrate every success no matter how big or small.

I know there will be days when it's all I can do to get out of bed, but on those days, I will celebrate the fact that I got out of bed.

Sunday

If you say, "Sadness is upon me." Instead of "I am Sad" then you aren't being the emotion it is a passing thing. And when it passes, some other feeling will be ON you for a while. I'm getting closer with this to figuring out how to label the situation I'm in with cancer.

Monday

Still waiting for the call for an appointment with the plastic surgeons. Hopefully tomorrow I will hear from them. But that doesn't make the waiting any easier. My Auntie told me (she's a retired RN) to expect to be completely laid up for two weeks after the surgery. ☹ I know it was going to be intense but *Two Weeks* of feeling like crap?!?!

Today has not been a good day. Hopefully tomorrow will have some answers and be better. The waiting is hard.

Wednesday

I try to be positive in my day-to-day dealings but when I am done and can let down my guard at home Grief and Anger, Sorrow and Rage are sitting at the table, waiting for me. "Come sit, we have things to say." So, I sit with them and listen to what they have to tell me. We move to chairs around the fireplace. In the same room where Cancer sat. The light is dim, the flickering of the flames illuminate our faces as I join them. I pull up my chair, closing the circle around the fire. The wood crackling and popping in the fireplace. The flagstone smooth beneath my feet, a drink warm in my hands, held for a future toast or to warm my frozen core. The room so different and yet the same.

Friday

My appointment with Plastics was on Tuesday. Today was a phone conversation with the Oncologist, Dr. Pete. The plastics appointment went really well. The surgeon, Dr. Johnson, was knowledgeable *and* had a sense of humor. He explained everything in as much detail as I wanted and didn't make me feel rushed. It was good but a bit surreal. Then came the phone appointment with Dr. Pete. It was to make sure I was happy with the plastic surgeon and the route I was taking with my surgery. But, somehow in my head, I was going to walk away with a date for the surgery. Almost had a full-on panic attack waiting for that call, and then, the doctor was late getting away from his hospital rounds. Thank goodness I had things at work to keep me busy until he called! But by the time he called, I felt like I was going to jump out of my skin. At the end of the 10 min call, he assured me that his office would work with Plastics' office and get a date set up and not to worry. It would be weeks not months away. In my head, *Weeks to wait to hear?* How on earth do people wait months to get a surgery date with this thing always hanging around? It's like a constant white noise that, at unexpected times, erupts into a racket. You know—just in case you forgot it was there. Like that'll happen. And so.... we wait.

Another Friday

A lot has happened, and I have been reading about Joy and how to use those slivers of joy to practice gratitude. It is hard to stay angry when you are being grateful for something.

Gratitude is something I started doing in a conscious way back in college. An assignment was to write five things you were thankful for each day for 30 days with no repeats. Not as easy as you'd think! Especially on the crappy days but so worth it; particularly on the crappy days.

In the midst of everything that has been happening to me, I have so much to be grateful for. Backing up here....

It had been almost a week of waiting. Seemed like longer and was really only day five. (I never know – is Wednesday five days from Friday or four?) I got the call from Dr. Pete's office that the surgery would be in exactly three weeks less a day. So, Tuesday. I told my manager and the two friends /coworkers who had been my closest supports through this and who would be most impacted by my being gone the news. I called my mom when I got home, and we talked about when she would come down and what I might need. I called my family and told them that we had a date, and I planned to see them the weekend before my surgery. I was so glad to have a date. Now, I could start preparing. Things that had to be done both at home and work now had an expiration date. Not just cleaning, freezing meals and such. I wanted to write letters to my kids and family to be delivered if something went wrong. This wasn't me being macabre. This was me looking after my family. I didn't expect anything to go wrong. I found comfort in being prepared. After I told my co-workers, I went back to my desk and worked really hard at not freaking out when all I really wanted to do was go home, throw myself across the bed like an angst-filled teen, and bawl. Because, while I was able to talk about the procedure, it was objective and 'just the facts, man,' I was a step removed from it. Now suddenly, the wrapping had been ripped off again, and all the emotions came roaring back to the surface, threatening to swamp me. So, I breathed deep and, picturing the feelings as a big fluorescent green blob, started shoving and squishing it back into the box. I shoved, pushed, squeezed, and almost pinched my fingers a few times closing the lid, but I got it shut. Then I sat on it like an overstuffed suitcase. Through the day it tried to escape, but I kept it in until I could be home. I may have shut it too tight, if my sleepless nights have been any measure. Standing guard all the time was exhausting! I felt like there was this solider guarding a solid room—no windows, just a tight-fitting door with a little slide window to check through. He was watching for escape attempts, and he was armed with a spear, so when any emotions tried to sneak out, he could jab it and make it retreat.

Monday

I had been learning how to let the emotions out a little at a time so they didn't get so full and big that they knocked down the door and flattened my poor guard. So, I sat at the table with them down here. A roughhewn table with a few wooden chairs. Not a comfortable room–warm enough, but stone floors and lights but no windows. I acknowledged the emotions—fear, grief, sorrow, anger, anxiety. But, at the table also sat relief, calmness, humbleness, acceptance, and gratefulness. As I recognized the upsetting emotions, I also had to acknowledge the positive ones.

Thursday

Mom came down. She will stay with me until I am back on my feet. I cannot express how glad I am to have her here. There is that one person who you turn to when things are going wrong. For me that is my mom. She is my strength when I am crumbling.

I got a package in the mail yesterday. I wasn't expecting anything, so it was exciting to see what I got. It was these wonderful stuffy hearts from the Women's Breast Health Clinic. They are for post-surgery to help and hold everything where it's supposed to be and be a cushion for the seatbelt. There was some more reading material in the package too but pulling those two pink hearts out of the bag? I felt so much caring in that moment holding those soft lovey hearts that someone had made by hand. People have said, 'Let me know how I can help."

And I have said this too. But I don't know how you can help, and I'm hesitant to ask. But this? These two little hearts? These said, "I know how to help. These are something you can use to help you feel better.' Now I know to say, I will make you some meals for the freezer. What kind of things do you like? Any allergies or hard no's? Okay, I'll bring them by on this day. Or do you need me to pick up prescriptions, groceries, books from the library, etc. This, for me, is huge, partly because I don't like cooking. So, on the days I'm not feeling up to it, I can take something out of the freezer and don't have to think. A phone call or text. A silly note, just because. An invite for a tea across town or a walk. A friend said they will make an extra plate and bring it over at supper. Another friend said she will bring me a pan of bran muffins to 'help things along.' The caring and support of my friends and family has filled my heart.

I am trying to live in the moment and not worry about what might happen. But it was very hard some days.

Handprints

No matter it's a passing glance and a smile to a stranger on the street.

The passionate embrace of a lover.

A handshake of a child's hug around your leg.

It can be a holding-a giving and taking of strength.

Holding each other up.

A strike in anger or a caress of affection.

A smile and a brush across an arm that says, "I see you."

Every encounter with another person leaves a mark behind.

We are all covered with the handprints of other people's touches in our lives.

Some we brush away, but others we tattoo on.

By A. Lady
April 2022

Doodles Go Here!

Surgery day, May 3

Not a date I'm likely to forget.

I have lines drawn all over the front of me. Marks so the surgeons will know where to cut and sew. Like setting a pattern on a piece of cloth. Except this pattern is on my skin in green marker. The staff are all very kind in their efficiency. They explain as they go—At least until I am unconscious. The hardest part of the day was watching my mom walk away down the hall when it was time to go into surgery. I wanted to call out to her to take me with her. I could tell she felt the same way.

In recovery

I woke up easy, and I was so relieved to be awake that I was unaware of anything else. No taking stock of my fingers and toes and everything in between. I was awake. That meant the surgery was done. My relief surpassed anything else. The cancer was gone. I didn't know how I knew this, but the same way I knew it was there before I was told and even which breast. I knew there was no cancer in me.

I had such a dry mouth! But no liquids yet until I woke up more. However, I got a sponge on a stick. I could dip it in my water and suck on it, as long as I didn't take in too much water, don't want to get sick. Never thought sucking on a sponge would be so wonderful! Ha-ha

The nurses came in every hour to check everything. They had a tiny ultrasound machine about the size of a deck of cards with a probe on it that they held under the flap (the dressing over the breast where the nipple used to be) and listened for the steady thump thump of the healthy, newly made vein. Then stiches, incisions, circulation and drains all got checked, along with blood pressure and stuff, so it did take a while. Every single hour. So, I slept when I could, took the pain &/or nausea medicine if I got the littlest twinge. Especially at first. The poor lady in the bed next to me threw up so much, even with extra medication. I couldn't imagine her pain, especially in her abs.

Standing and walking the first time after surgery was scary and exhausting and I felt like I had run a marathon walking the 10 feet to the bathroom. I was so happy to see my bed that I flopped down on it. No, not really. I crept to the edge of the bed and carefully sat down in a preplanned spot. As I *slowly* lowered myself onto my side the nurse lifted my legs to keep my core level. Then, slowly edged over onto my back where I needed to lay and pant for a moment before using my arms to pull myself up the rest of the way on the bed where I promptly fell into an exhausted sleep.

The first couple of times I sat on the toilet after they took the catheter out, I had to have a stern talking to my bladder. Sitting on the toilet; I'd look down at the *nothing happening* when it should have been automatic! Come on, pee already! Nothing. Really, you need to go; you're full. Nothing. Go Already! Still Nothing. Then finally, a little dribble. "YES! Like that! Do that more!" I cheered on my bladder. It finally remembered what to do and leisurely emptied itself. The next time was a little easier and quicker and with less coercing. Ha-ha

One night the Night RN and the Blood Pressure machine had a set to. She put the cuff on my arm, turned it on and it beeped at her. So, she reset some buttons and it beeped at her again. It sounded like an argument. Every time it started beeping at her, she would cut if off with beeps of her own, pushing the buttons. Made me laugh. You have to find fun in the little things.

Naps

They are wonderful things I have discovered. I don't know why child me fought them. I have learned to sleep every chance I get. My body is healing so much while I sleep. And I'm learning to take all the help I can get. I still need help with the most basic of things; like getting in and out of bed, getting dressed, changing my dressings and I don't feel like cooking or cleaning. I will pay it forward when it's my turn to help someone.

I got up for breakfast. Mom helped me change my dressings, then I'd have a nap. Wake up in time for lunch, go have a nap. Up again for dinner and then it was bedtime with one more dressing change first. I might have lain in bed and read until I was sleepy enough to sleep, but in bed I was.

The nurses in the hospital; and a friend after I was discharged, helped us put my belly band back on after a shower. Most wonderful shower was the first one after surgery—Even sitting on a stool. Had to keep my incisions as dry as possible for the first bit, so I just sat with my back to the water and leaned back to wash. So good to get the surgery off my skin and hair. The nurses at the hospital all raved about how beautiful the new breasts were. And there were two separate breasts. No uni-breast here! And they were impressive. Ha-ha. Like what they were in my early 20's, pre-children, life and gravity. Once everything has been done, I would have to get to know them. For the time being though, they were always in the bra except when I did my drains and checked on the incisions twice a day and that's too clinical. But I was so pleased that I went the route of getting it all done at once! I had nice boobs and a flatter stomach. I remember a conversation I had with a friend after I decided on the surgery. I joked with him that it was because of the cookies that I had enough tummy for them to do the re-construction. He laughed and said, "You will have *Cook-ie Boobs.*" That is what I have called them since too. It helps me to laugh.

The rewards outweighed the struggles in doing simple things. Like planning every move before I tried to get out of bed and calling for help when I was ready to move. It was like I was planning military maneuvers! If I put this leg here and my hand here....

Celebrate Every Victory. I cannot stress this enough. It has helped my healing and sanity. When I could use the bathroom by myself; pull up my pants all on my own? I celebrate the milestone in my healing. Celebrate with your tribe too. The first time I got out of and then back into bed by myself I did a little happy dance in my head. The things we all take for granted and suddenly I couldn't do were hard on my state of mind. But regaining that independence in inches felt so good. I have done a lot of mental and a few physical fist pumps celebrating my healing and getting back to my normal.

Even though I wore a belly band I still worked to tighten my abs. Just lying flat with a pillow under my knees and tightening my abs was a workout, but I didn't want them to be lazy either, depending on the band. Coughing and sneezing have still been a thing to watch out for, so I try and keep a pillow handy that I can roll up and hold against myself from abs to chest.

Change in and of itself isn't bad or good. It just is change. And bad and good things change to other bad and good things. So, Change is just different stuff taking the place of the current stuff.

I'm going to have to think about this. It makes sense but....

Thank goodness my mom was still there helping me. I was laying on the sofa, and when I rolled onto my side to sit up (a process in itself), I got stuck. I couldn't get my hand under me well enough to push myself up and I couldn't swing my legs over the edge to sit up because of my hand. And there I lay. After I got done laughing at the ridiculousness of it, I had Mom help me up. And I made sure I had a book or something to put under my hand on the sofa after that too!

Monday

Two weeks post-surgery I got my drains out (well three of them), and I could wear real clothes! Woo-Hoo! A loose t-shirt over yoga pants. (I brought them with me and changed before leaving the hospital) I was getting closer to being my normal self every day.

Tuesday

I got the news that I was officially cancer free. Mom came with me. I thought it was as important for the person closest to me to hear this from the doctor as it was me. I was excited and a little teary as I phoned the rest of my family to tell them.

Wednesday

Everything happened so fast that I hadn't had time to process any of my emotions. Sometime soon, I will have to, because otherwise, they play sneak attack and leak out at unexpected times.

I did my own dressing change, band, and bra today after my shower. I couldn't do them up on my own before now. Got dressed in regular clothes; t-shirt and pj pants since I was staying home. But the point is *I did it all myself!* Another step toward independence.

Another Tuesday

It had been six weeks since my surgery. I was mostly back to normal. Although, when I did overdo it, I was flat on my back for the next day and a half at least. *It's SO Frustrating!* I'm tired of being tired. I had to wear the support clothes (band and sports bra) all the time still. The only time they were off was for brief showers. The open areas under my breasts were almost closed. I had a couple of wire free bras coming. It was very hard to find wire free bras that weren't bralettes and I felt like I needed more support than they could give.

The sky was dark a moment ago, the rain pouring down. Then suddenly the sun was out. Everything was wet and dripping, but the sun was shining like it never happened. My emotions and thoughts were like that—Yo-Yoing up and down. I was fine, and suddenly I was swamped in tears; and then, was okay again.

Another day

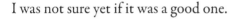

I was not sure yet if it was a good one.

There was cancer in my breast, and now there wasn't.

There wasn't cancer, and there wasn't a breast.

Oh, you wouldn't know it looking at me. There were breast shapes there, the form of them. The surgeon did an amazing job. And I was glad for them. But, looking at them reminded me of what I'd lost too. The lines of stiches. So carefully and beautifully done. The patchwork created an image of what used to be there. I was delighted and in awe of the medical science and skill behind what was done and still I grieved that it was necessary to happen. I was so thankful and so stricken at once. Cancer stole so much from me. And that it could have been so much worse, that it could have taken more if the thief hadn't been discovered so quickly, was a cold blanket I wrapped around myself searching for comfort.

If I ever have a lover, will he be repulsed by my lack of areoles and nipples and my scars? Because they all had to go—part of the milk duct. There was a circular scar where they would be. I could get nipple reconstruction and then the area tattooed to look closer to normal, I could leave it blank, or get something tattooed across them or even 3D nipples tattooed on. Lots of options which was great. Lots of ways to take back ownership and control of my body. Just like with the initial meeting with my cancer surgeon. He was able to give me options, and with my choices the plastic surgeon gave me more options too. I have been fortunate enough to feel like

I have had some control in this ride that has moved so fast. Like a car careening down a mountain road, and it took all of us to keep it on track and away from the cliffs. Not just the doctor and nurses either. I was so fortunate that my mom could come and stay with me for the first month. And the friends that called or texted often. Care packages and cards that made me laugh. Friends who dropped in to visit or phone that first four weeks to let me know they cared and to reassure me and themselves that I was still me and would be back with time.

And now, six weeks in, people were back at their lives, the crisis was past. And there was nothing to see here; I looked fine. But inside I felt jagged and sore. Tired. I had two more weeks to get myself together and go back to my job. And while I knew two weeks could make a huge difference, I still didn't know how I'd manage it. Just will I guess. Just like every other seemingly huge thing I've done. Just one step at a time. Just like the joke about how to eat an elephant—One bite at a time. And if that meant I had to take a nap at lunch or right after work? That was okay too.

Thursday

Well, so much for my brave words about taking naps and such. I just had a sneak attack from my body at noon. I had just plugged in the kettle for tea with my sandwich and suddenly I was dizzy, fuzzy brained and my eyes wanted to close right there. I've learned that this is my 'warning' that gives me about five minutes to lay down or fall down unconscious. I used to have these a lot right after surgery; but it had been weeks! Why today?

I was up again, lunch made and eaten; only two hours later. I still felt exhausted though. Maybe I could blame it on the grey rainy day. They always made good nap days. Maybe I'd take my lead weighted limbs back to bed again.

Saturday

It'd been four months now. Life as we knew it was back to normal.

I was so excited the other evening, I got to have a bath! Had to wait until the scaring was complete and no possible place for germs to get in. I needed to rub all the scars every day to keep them from sticking to the fascia layer below.

I still had appointments with my cancer doctor and plastic surgeon coming up in a couple of weeks. The cancer doctor to go over how the medication I'm on for the next five years was working for me. Some people get terrible side effects. And the plastic surgeon wanted to have one more look at how things were healing and discuss whether I was going to get the rest of the reconstruction surgery done. I was so fortunate. I had very little pain from my surgery, and the meds were not bothering me much at all. I got the odd hot flash, but not too big or long usually (and I was getting them before so, really). I had healed up wonderfully. There was some deeper scaring under the one breast but nothing you could see. And I mustn't forget my 'extra smile' ha-ha. But it was low enough that I could wear a bikini if I wanted.

Present Day

I am still working through stuff. I still have days when I am so angry and sad and grieving. There are good days too, when I get a compliment, or a friend calls to go for a tea across town, or I get to crunch through the fall leaves and feel the sun warm on my face. There are the times when I find a really good book and can sit and read it.

I have the support of my family and friends, and I see a wonderful counsellor when it gets too much, and she helps me untangle the ball of string that is my thoughts and emotions.

My doctor is helping me monitor and watch for signs of it sneaking back in. I have a wonderful group of people who are helping me stay on track and healthy both physically and mentally.

Cancer broke into my body. It was found in its hiding place and evicted.

There is a part of me that will always stand as a Sentinel. Always keeping watch.

There was cancer.

Now there is not.

A few tips I learned as I went that may help:

If you like your underwear, don't leave them on when you change into the hospital gown, even if the nurse says to. You will lose them, because when you are in surgery, they cut them off and toss them out. Can't put a catheter in with underwear in the way.

Sneezing/Coughing is a delicate process, and you have to move fast. If you have time, draw up the bottom of the bed so your knees are close without using your ab muscles to pull them towards you. Then, shove as much of the blankets into the space between your knees and stomach as you can, pull the pillow from behind your head and roll it in half and hug it to your chest and upper abs. Now, cough. I know it sounds like a process, but believe me, all it took was once of not doing this to never want to again.

Here's another fun fact. Your urine will be the most bilious shade of green if you had tracer dye injected for tracking the sentential lymph nodes. That's normal, but you want to push fluids, drink as much water as you can, once you can, and the IV fluids will do the rest. The nurse will want to pull the catheter soon. This is good because it is amazing how lazy and forgetful your bladder gets!

Take a sports bra with molded cups with you if you are getting reconstruction! One that fits your rib cage and is the right cup size you are going to be post-surgery. And most importantly – IT ZIPS UP IN THE FRONT! You cannot pull the bra over your head. The nurse will help you put this on as soon as possible after surgery. The compression of the molded cups will help with shaping and reduce swelling. Oh, did I feel better physically and mentally after getting the girls tucked in tight. There is a camisole you can get if you are not getting reconstruction done. But an inexpensive sports bra is the way to go for reconstruction. It will be stained from your healing incisions and drains so you will probably want to throw it away after. Also, get some men's PJs with the button up shirt and draw string pants. They are loose and roomy, open in the front, and if you put a sweater over them, you can wear them out. There is room for your grenades (the drains that are pinned to your belly band) inside the pants, and with a long sweater no one will notice the strange bulges in your pants. Yoga pants are too tight for the drains.

Eat fresh prunes, bran muffins, raw vegies, and drink lots of water. I was lucky; a friend brought me over a big pan of raisin bran muffins. So that was breakfast solved! Whatever works so you don't get constipated. The pain killers cause constipation, and you don't want your poor abs to work harder than they already are or pull your incision! The nurse told me I have an extra smile now—from hip bone to hip bone. ☺

If you have a tall bed (as in higher than your butt can sit straight down on), get a step stool. I used a little single step kitchen stool. I can step up onto it, turn and sit and then, with help, lay down. Also, when you push up on the mattress as your legs get lifted over the edge of the bed it's difficult because mattresses are soft. But if you put a book under your pushing up hand? Wow, what a difference! The stability and your hand not sinking into the bed? Amazing. Works good on the sofa too. Ha-ha

There are lots of resources out there, both online and in print. There are books at the public libraries, and your doctor will be able to suggest good, reliable places to find information. Please don't use "Dr. Google" to find resources.

You will get through this. You will find your strength in unexpected places and support everywhere. Talk to your family, friends, pastor, co-workers, counsellor about what is happening as long as you feel safe and comfortable talking with them. Don't share more than you are comfortable with. And if someone asks invasive questions, instead of telling them what they want, ask "Why do you want to know?" It usually stops the nosey questions in their tracks.

Remember, you are not alone. There have been many women who have been in the chair where you now sit. And even though you can't see us, we all are there supporting you.

Printed in the USA
CPSIA information can be obtained
at www.ICGtesting.com
JSHW010751110224
57066JS00011B/210